CW01044776

Contents

INTRODUCTION

For the organ without any purpose, appendix causes its share of problems. It is one of the most common emergency surgery performed. After the important surgery, it is imperative to follow a proper Appendicitis diet. Appendicitis diet should primarily include Vitamin A, Vitamin C, Zinc, Omega-3 fatty acids, glutamine, etc. The healthy liver function should be maintained in order to have a faster recovery.

Boosting immune system after the surgery is important. Your body should not avoid taking any nutrients. At this time, your body is prone to the

4

infection and demands proper healing. Vitamin C rich food such as orange, guava, lemon, etc. can be very useful in this condition. An extra zinc supplement can also be taken with zinc-rich food. Carrots and sweet potatoes which are good sources of Vitamin A should be consumed along with the other food. Vitamin D is important to have a healthy body, high-quality supplements of which include eggs, fish, cheese, ginger, etc.

A highly liquid diet such as juices and beverages are recommended to have an easy digestion. Fiber should also be included on your plate. Generally, it is advised to consume the soft food during this period. The patient should not take this condition lightly and follow the diet

accordingly.

APPENDICITIS

An excruciating pain in the lower right abdomen

is generally (read fearfully) construed as

appendicitis, which is characterized by the

painful inflammation of the appendix.

Appendicitis is a clinical emergency, and in the

case of any negligence it may get complicated

and cause serious infections, or worse, prove

fatal.

If left untreated, appendicitis can cause your

appendix to burst. This can cause bacteria to spill

into your abdominal cavity, which can be serious and sometimes fatal.

APPENDICITIS SYMPTOMS

If you have appendicitis, you may experience one or more of the following symptoms:

• pain in your upper abdomen or around your bellybutton

• pain in the lower right side of your abdomen

• loss of appetite

• indigestion

• nausea

• vomiting

- diarrhea

- constipation

- abdominal swelling

- inability to pass gas

- low-grade fever

Appendicitis pain may start off as mild cramping. It often becomes more steady and severe over time. It may start in your upper abdomen or bellybutton area, before moving to the lower right quadrant of your abdomen.

If you're constipated and you suspect that you may have appendicitis, avoid taking laxatives or using an enema. These treatments may cause your appendix to burst.

Contact your doctor if you have tenderness in the right side of your abdomen along with any of other symptoms of appendicitis. Appendicitis can quickly become a medical emergency. Get the information you need to recognize this serious condition.

APPENDICITIS CAUSES

In many cases, the exact cause of appendicitis is unknown. Experts believe it develops when part of the appendix becomes obstructed, or blocked.

Many things can potentially block your appendix, including:

- a buildup of hardened stool

- enlarged lymphoid follicles

- intestinal worms

- traumatic injury

- tumors

When your appendix becomes blocked, bacteria can multiply inside it. This can lead to the formation of pus and swelling, which can cause painful pressure in your abdomen.

Other conditions can also cause abdominal pain.

Click here to read about other potential causes of

pain in your lower right abdomen.

RISK FACTORS FOR APPENDICITIS

Appendicitis can affect anyone. But some people

may be more likely to develop this condition than

others. For example, risk factors for appendicitis

include:

• Age: Appendicitis most often affects people

between the ages of 15 and 30 years old.

• Sex: Appendicitis is more common in males

than females.

• Family history: People who have a family history of appendicitis are at heightened risk of developing it.

Although more research is needed, low-fiber diets might also raise the risk of appendicitis.

TYPES OF APPENDICITIS

Appendicitis can be acute or chronic. In acute cases of appendicitis, the symptoms tend to be severe and develop suddenly. In chronic cases, the symptoms may be milder and may come and go over several weeks, months, or even years.

The condition can also be simple or complex. In simple cases of appendicitis, there are no complications. Complex cases involve

complications, such as an abscess or ruptured

appendix.

TESTS FOR APPENDICITIS

If your doctor suspects you might have

appendicitis, they will perform a physical exam.

They will check for tenderness in the lower right

part of your abdomen and swelling or rigidity.

Depending on the results of your physical exam,

your doctor may order one or more tests to

check for signs of appendicitis or rule out other

potential causes of your symptoms.

There's no single test available to diagnose appendicitis. If your doctor can't identify any other causes of your symptoms, they may diagnose the cause as appendicitis.

Complete blood count

To check for signs of infection, your doctor may order a complete blood count (CBC). To conduct this test, they will collect a sample of your blood and send it to a lab for analysis.

Appendicitis is often accompanied by bacterial infection. An infection in your urinary tract or other abdominal organs may also cause symptoms similar to those of appendicitis.

Urine tests

To rule out urinary tract infection or kidney stones as a potential cause of your symptoms, your doctor may use urinalysis. This is also known as a urine test.

Your doctor will collect a sample of your urine that will be examined in a lab.

Pregnancy test

Ectopic pregnancy can be mistaken for appendicitis. It happens when a fertilized egg implants itself in a fallopian tube, rather than the uterus. This can be a medical emergency.

If your doctor suspects you might have an ectopic pregnancy, they may perform a pregnancy test. To conduct this test, they will collect a sample of your urine or blood. They may also use a transvaginal ultrasound to learn where the fertilized egg has implanted.

Pelvic exam

If you're female, your symptoms might be caused by pelvic inflammatory disease, an ovarian cyst, or another condition affecting your reproductive organs.

To examine your reproductive organs, your doctor may perform a pelvic exam.

During this exam, they will visually inspect your vagina, vulva, and cervix. They will also manually inspect your uterus and ovaries. They may collect a sample of tissue for testing.

Abdominal imaging tests

To check for inflammation of your appendix, your doctor might order imaging tests of your abdomen. This can also help them identify other potential causes of your symptoms, such as an abdominal abscess or fecal impaction.

Your doctor may order one or more of the following imaging tests:

• abdominal ultrasound

- abdominal X-ray

- abdominal CT scan

- abdominal MRI scan

In some cases, you might need to stop eating food for a period of time before your test. Your doctor can help you learn how to prepare for it.

Chest imaging tests

Pneumonia in the lower right lobe of your lungs can also cause symptoms similar to appendicitis.

If your doctor thinks you might have pneumonia, they will likely order a chest X-ray. They may also order a CT scan to create detailed images of your lungs.

CAN YOUR DOCTOR USE AN ULTRASOUND TO DIAGNOSE APPENDICITIS?

If your doctor suspects you might have appendicitis, they may order an abdominal ultrasound. This imaging test can help them check for signs of inflammation, an abscess, or other problems with your appendix.

Your doctor may order other imaging tests as well. For example, they may order a CT scan. An ultrasound uses high frequency sound waves to create pictures of your organs, while a CT scan uses radiation.

Compared to an ultrasound, a CT scan creates more detailed images of your organs. However, there are some health risks associated with radiation exposure from a CT scan. Your doctor can help you understand the potential benefits and risks of different imaging test.

TREATMENT OPTIONS FOR APPENDICITIS

Depending on your condition, your doctor's recommended treatment plan for appendicitis may include one or more of the following:

• surgery to remove your appendix

• needle drainage or surgery to drain an abscess

• antibiotics

• pain relievers

• IV fluids

• liquid diet

In rare cases, appendicitis may get better without surgery. But in most cases, you will need surgery to remove your appendix. This is known as an appendectomy.

If you have an abscess that hasn't ruptured, your doctor may treat the abscess before you undergo surgery. To start, they will give you antibiotics. Then they will use a needle to drain the abscess of pus.

SURGERY FOR APPENDICITIS

To treat appendicitis, your doctor may use a type

of surgery known as appendectomy. During this

procedure, they will remove your appendix. If

your appendix has burst, they will also clean out

your abdominal cavity.

In some cases, your doctor may use laparoscopy

to perform minimally invasive surgery. In other

cases, they may have to use open surgery to

remove your appendix.

Like any surgery, there are some risks associated

with appendectomy. However, the risks of

appendectomy are smaller than the risks of

untreated appendicitis. Find out more about the

potential risks and benefits of this surgery.

Acute appendicitis

Acute appendicitis is a severe and sudden case of appendicitis. The symptoms tend to develop quickly over the course of one to two days.

It requires immediate medical treatment. If left untreated, it can cause your appendix to rupture. This can be a serious and even fatal complication.

Acute appendicitis is more common than chronic appendicitis. Learn more about the similarities and differences between these conditions.

Chronic appendicitis

Chronic appendicitis is less common than acute appendicitis. In chronic cases of appendicitis, the symptoms may be relatively mild. They may disappear before reappearing again over a period of weeks, months, or even years.

This type of appendicitis can be challenging to diagnose. Sometimes, it's not diagnosed until it develops into acute appendicitis.

Chronic appendicitis can be dangerous. Get the information you need to recognize and treat this condition.

APPENDICITIS IN KIDS

An estimated 70,000 children experience appendicitis every year in the United States. Although it's most common in people between the ages of 15 and 30 years old, it can develop at any age.

In children and teenagers, appendicitis often causes a stomachache near the navel. This pain may eventually become more severe and move to the lower right side of your child's abdomen.

Your child may also:

• lose their appetite

• develop a fever

• feel nauseous

• vomit

If your child develops symptoms of appendicitis, contact their doctor right away. Learn why it's so important to get treatment.

RECOVERY TIME FOR APPENDICITIS

Your recovery time for appendicitis will depend on multiple factors, including:

• your overall health

• whether or not you develop complications from appendicitis or surgery

• the specific type of treatments you receive

If you have laparoscopic surgery to remove your appendix, you may be discharged from the hospital a few hours after you finish surgery or the next day.

If you have open surgery, you will likely need to spend more time in the hospital to recover afterward. Open surgery is more invasive than laparoscopic surgery and typically requires more follow-up care.

Before you leave the hospital, your healthcare provider can help you learn how to care for your incision sites. They may prescribe antibiotics or pain relievers to support your recovery process. They may also advise you to adjust your diet, avoid strenuous activity, or make other changes to your daily habits while you heal.

It may take several weeks for you to fully recover from appendicitis and surgery. If you develop complications, your recovery may take longer. Learn about some of the strategies you can use to promote a full recovery.

APPENDICITIS IN PREGNANCY

Acute appendicitis is the most common non-obstetric emergency requiring surgery during pregnancy. It affects an estimated 0.04 to 0.2 percent of pregnant women.

The symptoms of appendicitis may be mistaken for routine discomfort from pregnancy.

Pregnancy may also cause your appendix to shift upward in your abdomen, which can affect the location of appendicitis-related pain. This can make it harder to diagnose.

Treatment options during pregnancy might include one or more of the following:

• surgery to remove your appendix

• needle drainage or surgery to drain an abscess

• antibiotics

Delayed diagnosis and treatment may increase your risk of complications, including miscarriage.

Potential complications of appendicitis

Appendicitis can cause serious complications. For example, it may cause a pocket of pus known as an abscess to form in your appendix. This abscess may leak pus and bacteria into your abdominal cavity.

Appendicitis can also lead to a ruptured appendix. If your appendix ruptures, it can spill fecal matter and bacteria into your abdominal cavity.

If bacteria spill into your abdominal cavity, it can cause the lining of your abdominal cavity to become infected and inflamed. This is known as peritonitis, and it can be very serious, even fatal.

Bacterial infections can also affect other organs in your abdomen. For example, bacteria from a ruptured abscess or appendix may enter your bladder or colon. It may also travel through your bloodstream to other parts of your body.

To prevent or manage these complications, your doctor may prescribe antibiotics, surgery, or other treatments. In some cases, you might develop side effects or complications from treatment. However, the risks associated with antibiotics and surgery tend to be less serious than the potential complications of untreated appendicitis.

PREVENTING APPENDICITIS

There's no sure way to prevent appendicitis. But you might be able to lower your risk of developing it by eating a fiber-rich diet. Although more research is needed on the potential role of diet, appendicitis is less common in countries where people eat high-fiber diets.

Foods that are high in fiber include:

• fruits

• vegetables

• lentils, split peas, beans, and other legumes

• oatmeal, brown rice, whole wheat, and other whole grains

Your doctor may also encourage you to take a

fiber supplement.

Add fiber by

• sprinkling oat bran or wheat germ over

breakfast cereals, yogurt, and salads

• cooking or baking with whole-wheat flour

whenever possible

• swapping white rice for brown rice

• adding kidney beans or other legumes to salads

• eating fresh fruit for dessert

APPENDICITIS AND HOME REMEDIES

Contact your doctor right away if you experience symptoms of appendicitis. It's a serious condition that requires medical treatment. And it's not safe to rely on home remedies to treat it.

If you undergo surgery to remove your appendix, your doctor may prescribe antibiotics and pain relievers to support your recovery. In addition to taking medications as prescribed, it may help to:

• get lots of rest

• drink plenty of fluids

• go for a gentle walk each day

• avoid strenuous activity and lifting heavy objects until your doctor says it's safe to do so

• keep your surgical incision sites clean and dry

In some cases, your doctor might encourage you to adjust your diet. If you're feeling nauseous after surgery, it might help to eat bland foods such as toast and plain rice. If you're constipated, it might help to take a fiber supplement.

HOW TO PREVENT AND TREAT APPENDICITIS NATURALLY?

Although self-medication isn't advisable for appendicitis, some natural remedies can help in subduing the chances of its occurrence and may help alleviate the pain. Here are the remedies to manage appendicitis naturally:

1. Fenugreek Seeds

Fenugreek seeds aid in preventing the formation of mucus and pus inside the appendix and thereby ease the acute abdominal pain.

How to consume: Boil two tablespoons of fenugreek seeds in one liter of water for about half an hour. Strain the water and consume it twice a day until the symptoms of appendicitis start to subside.

2. Mint

Mint is useful to soothe the symptoms of appendicitis, such as nausea, vomiting.

How to consume: Prepare mint tea by boiling few mint leaves in water. This can be taken thrice daily to get relief from the appendix pain.

3. Buttermilk

Buttermilk is beneficial in appendicitis, as it is light to digest. It also offers essential probiotics that help in mitigating the growth of the bacteria or any infection.

How to consume: In a glass of buttermilk add grated cucumber, ginger, crushed mint, and coriander leaves with a pinch of salt. This refreshing drink can be taken throughout the day. You can also consume buttermilk as is.

4. Green Grams

Considered an age-old remedy, green grams are a highly nutritive eating option. They contain anti-inflammatory compounds.

How to consume: Soak green grams in water overnight and consume them the next day raw, steamed or sautéed (in the form of salad). You can have it three times a day to keep the abdomen pain away.

5. Garlic

Garlic has antibacterial and anti-inflammatory properties. These properties make it an effective option against appendicitis.

How to consume: You can crush a few garlic cloves and consume it with water. You can also choose to have garlic tablets. It is advisable to consume garlic on an empty stomach.

APPENDICITIS DIET

For the organ without any purpose, appendix causes its share of problems. It is one of the most common emergency surgery performed. After the important surgery, it is imperative to follow a proper Appendicitis diet. Appendicitis diet should primarily include Vitamin A, Vitamin C, Zinc, Omega-3 fatty acids, glutamine, etc. The healthy liver function should be maintained in order to have a faster recovery.

Boosting immune system after the surgery is important. Your body should not avoid taking any nutrients. At this time, your body is prone to the infection and demands proper healing. Vitamin C rich food such as orange, guava, lemon, etc. can be very useful in this condition. An extra zinc supplement can also be taken with zinc-rich food. Carrots and sweet potatoes which are good sources of Vitamin A should be consumed along with the other food. Vitamin D is important to have a healthy body, high-quality supplements of which include eggs, fish, cheese, ginger, etc.

A highly liquid diet such as juices and beverages are recommended to have an easy digestion. Fiber should also be included on your plate. Generally, it is advised to consume the soft food during this period. The patient should not take this condition lightly and follow the diet accordingly.

FOOD ITEMS TO AVOID

Consumption of high-fat food is a strict no-no if you have appendicitis or in the post-surgery period, as these foods are difficult to digest.

High-fat food contains meat, cooked egg, cheese, whole mik, chocolate, ice cream, fried foods and preparations having high butter and oil.

• Food with high sugar content like sweets, candy, cake, muffins, sweeteners, ice cream, etc.

• Canned foods and juices

• Aerated drinks

• Beverages

• Alcohol

• Pepper and spices

• Condiments

• Beans and cruciferous vegetables that form gas

• Bakery items that contain cereal and white flour

DO'S AND DONT'S

• Low enemas, containing about one pint (1/2litre) of warm water should be administered every day for the first three days to cleanse the lower bowel.

• Hot compresses may be placed over the painful area several times daily.

• Abdominal packs, made of a strip of wet sheet covered by a dry flannel cloth bound tightly around the abdomen, should be applied continuously until all acute symptoms subside.

43

• After spending three days on fruit juices the patient may adopt 'an all-fruit diet for a further four or five days. During this period he should have three meals a day of fresh juicy fruits.

• Thereafter he should adopt a well balanced diet based on three basic food groups namely seeds nuts and grains vegetables and fruits.

• Certain vegetable juices especially carrot juice in combination with the juices of beets and cucumbers have been found valuable in the treatment of appendicitis.

• Regular use of tea made from fenugreek seeds has also proved helpful. In preventing the appendix from becoming a dumping ground for excess mucous and intestinal waste.

FOOD ITEMS YOU CAN EASILY CONSUME

• Fresh lime squeezed in lukewarm water and mixed with honey (one teaspoon) after getting up in the morning.

• Fruits and milk for breakfast along with some nuts, if required. A full milk diet is also good for an appendicitis patient, though it has to be seen whether he/she is being able to take it without having a problem.

• Steamed vegetables and buttermilk for lunch. May be a whole-wheat tortilla can be added.

• Fresh fruit or vegetable juice in the afternoon.

• Fresh vegetable salad, sprouted seeds, homemade cheese and buttermilk for dinner.

• Juice of carrot, cucumber and beet really helps an appendicitis patient.

• Tea made from fenugreek seeds also gives a soothing effect.

FOODS TO BE TAKEN

• A high fibre diet full of fresh fruits and green leafy vegetables is the best way to avoid this condition

• Beetroot, carrot and cucumber juices are all very helpful in naturally preventing and treating appendicitis

• Small quantities of green gram consumed thrice every day is a useful treatment for acute appendicitis

• Simple recipes like brown rice with vegetables such as green peppers, broccoli, cauliflower, beans and peas are easy to digest and are high in fibre which is very beneficial to appendicitis patients. Other preparations like chicken soup and steamed vegetable salads are also very good for recovering patients.

• Whole wheat including wheat germ and bran should be consumed regularly to avoid appendicitis and various other digestive ailments

• Chronic appendicitis can also be treated by consuming a liter of buttermilk every day.

DIET AFTER APPENDICITIS

Having an infection in your appendix, known as appendicitis, doesn't always require surgery. If your appendicitis is mild, your physician might give you antibiotics and tell you to follow a liquid or soft-foods diet. Even if your symptoms progress and you undergo surgery, which is an appendectomy, you'll likely have the same dietary requirements -- liquid or soft foods.

These diets are low in fiber and easy for your

body to digest. Follow your doctor's instructions

carefully. Normally you can get back to your

regular diet within a week or two, or as

tolerated.

Full-Liquid Diet

If you're feeling nauseated or have severe pain,

the thought of eating solid foods probably

doesn't appeal to you. But you still need to get

some nutrients into your system to help you

heal. A full-liquid diet allows you to consume just

about anything you want in liquid form, or foods

that would be liquid at room temperature. Drink

any kind of beverages: milk, juice, water or diet

soda. You can typically have coffee or tea, but

the caffeine might keep you awake, and you

need your rest. Consider drinking nutritional

shakes or liquid supplements -- either premade

or homemade smoothies -- to sneak in more

vitamins, minerals and even protein. Also enjoy

ice cream, frozen yogurt, gelatin, frozen pops,

pudding, custard or strained soups.

Soft-Foods Diet

Usually you can move up to the soft-foods diet

after you've been on a full-liquid diet for a few

days with no complications. This type of diet

allows you to gradually start adding fibrous foods

back into your system. In addition to everything

allowed in the full-liquid diet, you can also add in

cheese or yogurt. You can have small portions of

lean proteins, such as poultry, seafood, eggs and

fish. Enjoy fruits and vegetables without skins

sparingly. Things like mashed potatoes, canned

fruits, applesauce, avocados and tomato

products are generally well-tolerated. Have white

bread, cereal, biscuits, pancakes, crackers or

waffles, too. However, avoid whole-grain

varieties at this time to keep your fiber intake

down and allow your digestive tract to heal.

When to Get More Fiber

If you're on pain medications to manage your appendicitis, you can quickly become constipated. Your doctor may recommend eating certain easy-to-digest foods to up your fiber intake slightly. Add berries to smoothies, have a baked potato with the skin on or make a batch of beans -- soak them overnight to remove some of the carbohydrates that make you gassy. While you're healing, gradually work your way up to getting 100 percent of the daily value of fiber: 25 grams a day. Nutrition facts labels on packaged foods should clearly list the fiber grams for you.

7 DAYS MEAL ROASTER FOR APPENDICITIS DIET

Sunday

Breakfast (8:00-8:30AM)   1 cup of oats
and milk porridge

Mid-Meal (11:00-11:30AM)   1 glass tender
coconut water

Lunch (2:00-2:30PM)   1 cup broken
wheat porridge

Evening (4:00-4:30PM)   1 glass
buttermilk

Dinner (8:00-8:30PM)   1 cup rice
porridge

Monday

Breakfast (8:00-8:30AM)   1 cup of dalia

porridge

Mid-Meal (11:00-11:30AM)   1 glass tender

coconut water

Lunch (2:00-2:30PM)   1 cup cooked

vegetables (except beans, cruciferous

vegetables)

Evening (4:00-4:30PM)   1 glass carrot

juice

Dinner (8:00-8:30PM)   1 cup rawa

porridge

Tuesday

Breakfast (8:00-8:30AM)   1 cup of sago
porridge

Mid-Meal (11:00-11:30AM)   1 glass tender
coconut water

Lunch (2:00-2:30PM)   1 cup boiled
carrot with white rice

Evening (4:00-4:30PM)   1 cup moong
dal water

Dinner (8:00-8:30PM) 1 cup ragi porridge with
buttermilk

Wednesday

Breakfast (8:00-8:30AM)   2 aappam

with 1 tsp mild coconut chutney

Mid-Meal (11:00-11:30AM)   1 glass tender

coconut water

Lunch (2:00-2:30PM)   1 cup of

white rice with boilled vegetables (bhindi, snake

gourd and bottle gourd)

Evening (4:00-4:30PM)   1 stewed

apple with out skin

Dinner (8:00-8:30PM)   1 cup barley

porridge with buttermilk

Thursday

Breakfast (8:00-8:30AM)   2 idly with 1

tsp of mild tomato chutney

Mid-Meal (11:00-11:30AM)   1 glass tender

coconut water

Lunch (2:00-2:30PM)   1 cup well

cooked red gram dal and white rice

Evening (4:00-4:30PM)   1 glass barley

water

Dinner (8:00-8:30PM)   1 cup boiled

carrot and cucumber

Friday

Breakfast (8:00-8:30AM)   2 dosa with 1

tsp of mild mint chutney

Mid-Meal (11:00-11:30AM)   1 glass tender

coconut water

Lunch (2:00-2:30PM)   1 cup of well

cooked moong dal with white rice

Evening (4:00-4:30PM)   1 glass of

cucumber juice

Dinner (8:00-8:30PM)   1 cup of fruit

salad (apple with out skin, papaya, musk melon)

Saturday

Breakfast (8:00-8:30AM)   1 cup of rawa

upma

Mid-Meal (11:00-11:30AM)   1 glass tender

coconut water

Lunch (2:00-2:30PM)   1 cup of

white rice with 1/2 cup of boilled vegetables

(carrot, beet root and yellow cucumber)

Evening (4:00-4:30PM)   1 cup clear

chicken soup

Dinner (8:00-8:30PM)   1 cup oats

porridge

CONCLUSION

After your phases of consuming only liquids and soft foods, start adding other foods you like back into your diet, but not until your doctor advises you to do so. Don't dive right back into your old ways as soon as you get the green light -- you don't want to make yourself sick. Start with just a typical breakfast or lunch for a few days. Then as long as you don't have any side effects, start adding back your snacks. Whether you're recovering from appendicitis with or without surgery, you shouldn't have any longstanding dietary restrictions.

Printed in Great Britain
by Amazon

40839271R00036